D1413116

THE DASH DIET FOR BEGINNERS

A Quick Start Guide to Fast Natural Weight Loss, Lower Blood Pressure and Better Health with the DASH Diet, Including a 7-Day Meal Plan

Gina Crawford

© Copyright

Table of Contents

Introduction

Chapter 1 - What is the DASH diet?

Chapter 2 -Why was the DASH diet created?

Chapter 3 - Characteristics of the DASH Diet

Chapter 4 - DASH Diet Food Groups

Chapter 5 - Portion Control and Serving Sizes

Chapter 6 - DASH Diet Food List

Chapter 7 - The DASH diet and Weight Loss

Chapter 8 - Tips to Make the Switch to DASH Diet Eating

Chapter 9 - Tips to Lower Your Sodium Intake

Chapter 10 - DASH Diet Seven-Day Meal Plan

Chapter 11 - DASH Diet 30 Minute Recipes

   Raspberry Muffins

   Buckwheat Pancakes

   Sun-Dried Tomato Basil Pizza

   Chicken in White Wine and Mushroom Sauce

Balsamic Chicken Salad with Pineapple

Roasted Salmon with Chives and Tarragon

Triple Berry Spinach Salad

Simple Mango Salad

Tomato Basil Bruschetta

Fruit Kebabs with Lemony Lime Dip

Artichoke Dip

Peach Honey Spread

Conclusion

Introduction

The DASH diet is a lifelong well-balanced approach to healthy eating promoted by the National Institutes of Health that is based on nutrient-rich whole foods.

This book will teach you exactly how to reach and maintain a healthy weight while lowering blood pressure and cholesterol.

U.S News and World Report chose the DASH diet as the best overall diet, the healthiest diet and the best diet for diabetes for four years in a row.

It is estimated that hypertension or high blood pressure affects over one billion people worldwide. Not only is high blood pressure the leading cause of death, it also increases the risk of stroke and heart disease.

The DASH diet seeks to reduce sodium in your diet and increase your consumption of calcium, magnesium, potassium and fiber by eating a wide selection of whole foods that lower blood pressure.

Eating vegetables, fruits, whole grains, fish, lean meats, low fat dairy and healthy fats is all part of the DASH diet healthy eating plan.

The DASH diet is endorsed by the American Heart Association and is scientifically proven to lower blood pressure and cholesterol. Research has also shown that the DASH diet is extremely effective in promoting weight loss which has popularized it as a weight loss diet.

In a step-by-step way *The DASH Diet for Beginners Quick Start Guide* is going to teach you everything you need to know about how to successfully apply the DASH diet to your life!

Chapter 1
What is the DASH diet?

"Let food be thy medicine and medicine be thy food"
Hippocrates

The DASH diet is a well-balanced, lifelong approach to healthy eating that was discovered in research funded by the National Institutes of Health (NIH) to determine the role of dietary eating patterns on blood pressure.

Over the years a number of studies have proven that the DASH diet is not only effective for lowering blood pressure through diet but it is also effective in reducing the risk of cardiovascular disease, several types of cancers, stroke, heart disease, kidney stones, kidney disease, diabetes, heart failure and many other diseases.

The DASH diet has also been shown to promote weight loss and improve overall health.

The Dash diet is recommended by:

The Mayo Clinic

That American Heart Association

The American College of Cardiology

The Dietary Guidelines for Americans

US guidelines for the treatment of hypertension

The National Heart, Lung and Blood Institute (a part of the National Institutes of Health [NIH] of the US Dept of Health & Human Services)

The best overall diet

In January 2014 US News and World Report selected the DASH diet as the best overall diet, the healthiest diet and the best diet for diabetes for four years in a row.

The DASH diet was chosen by a distinguished panel of doctors for its healthy balance of food groups, its ability to improve health and its proven track record of successfully working time and time again.

Chapter 2

Why was the Dash diet created?

DASH stands for Dietary Approaches to Stop Hypertension. Hypertension or high blood pressure has been on the rise in the US for the past 50 years.

The continued increase of hypertension led the National Institutes of Health to propose funding for research that would study the impact of dietary patterns on blood pressure.

In 1992, the National Heart, Lung and Blood Institute worked closely with five prestigious medical research centers in the US to design and carry out the largest and most detailed study ever conducted called "The DASH study."

The DASH study was uniquely based on foods that the average person could buy at a local grocery store thus making it easy for anyone to implement.

The DASH study

The first DASH study began in 1993 and ended in July 1997. The study compared two experimental diets with one control diet. Each of the 459 screened participants were randomly selected to participate in one of three groups. They were instructed to follow the dietary pattern of that group for eight weeks in which time their blood pressure would be regularly checked.

The two experimental groups included:

Experimental diet group 1

Fruits and vegetables diet

Other than a high consumption of fruits and vegetables, this group was to eat the typical American diet with fewer sweets and snacks. Their fiber content was high and their magnesium and potassium levels were similar to 75% of people in the US.

Experimental diet group 2

The DASH diet

This group was to consume a high intake of fruits, vegetables and low-fat dairy. Fat content was low and protein and fiber levels were high. This diet was rich in magnesium, potassium, calcium, fish, poultry, whole grains and nuts. The consumption of red meats, sweets and sweetened drinks was low.

This diet intentionally included foods that would reduce blood pressure. It also contained a lot of antioxidant rich foods.

Control group

The Control diet

This group was to consume food that was typical of the American diet: low in potassium, calcium, fiber and magnesium and high in protein and fat.

The results of the DASH study

The results of the DASH study proved that dietary patterns *do* affect people with moderate to severe hypertension.

The fruits and vegetables group experienced lower blood pressure but their decrease was not as significant as the DASH group.

The participants in the DASH group that did not have hypertension experienced a decrease in blood pressure as well.

The study also showed that people with hypertension in the DASH diet group experienced a decrease in their blood pressure within only two weeks of starting the DASH diet.

The DASH sodium study

The second DASH study called "The DASH sodium study" was undertaken following "The DASH study" to see whether the DASH diet could lower blood pressure even more effectively if it were low in salt.

The two main objectives of the The DASH sodium study were:

To study the effects of reduced sodium levels on the DASH diet

To study the effects of the DASH diet at three different sodium levels

The DASH sodium study was a large scale study that ran from 1997 to 1999. It involved 412 adult participants with stage 1 hypertension or prehypertension. There were two groups involved:

The DASH diet group

The typical American diet group (the control diet group)

Each group was given a 30 day diet that included three different sodium levels: 3000 mg, 2400 mg and 1500 mg a day. Each diet was preceded by two weeks of high sodium control diet eating followed by 30 days of eating an assigned diet that randomized the sodium levels.

The results of the DASH sodium study

Both the DASH diet and the control diet were successful at lowering blood pressure at the lower salt levels but the biggest decrease in blood pressure was seen when the DASH diet was combined with low salt consumption of 1500 mg a day.

The results of this study also led researchers to propose that the national daily allowance of sodium be lowered.

The U.S. Dietary Guidelines for Americans recommend 2300 mg of sodium per day or lower. 1500 mg of sodium a day is recommended for people who have high blood pressure.

Chapter 3

Characteristics of the DASH Diet

The DASH diet is not necessarily a "diet" rather it is a way of eating that will promote long term health. The USDA (U.S. Department of Agriculture) recommends the DASH diet as "an ideal eating plan for all Americans."

The NIH (National Institutes of Health) says that the DASH diet plan does more than promote good eating habits, it offers suggestions on healthy alternatives to junk food and processed food.

In addition to this, the creators of the DASH diet have said... "not only is the DASH diet designed to bring down high blood pressure, it is also a well-balanced approach to eating that encourages people to lower their intake of sodium (salt) and increase their consumption of calcium, magnesium and potassium."

The characteristics of the DASH diet include:

Lower sodium intake

Increased vitamins and minerals

Increased good fats

Increased fiber consumption

Reduction of alcohol and caffeine

Customizable sodium and caloric intake

Lower sodium intake

The DASH diet provides guidelines for your sodium and caloric intake.

The standard DASH diet allows up to a maximum of 2300 mg of sodium per day and the low-sodium version of the DASH diet allows up to 1500 mg of sodium per day.

The average American diet contains up to 3500 mg of sodium per day.

Increased vitamins and minerals

All your essential vitamins and minerals are provided on the DASH diet by the many fruits, vegetables, whole grains and other whole foods that you are encouraged to eat on the diet.

The diet also includes an ample supply of minerals like magnesium and potassium that help to lower or improve your blood pressure.

Increased good fats

Consuming a lot of good fats and minimizing bad fats is highly encouraged on the DASH diet. Saturated and Trans fats should be replaced with lean meats, omega-3's from fish and seafood, low-fat dairy, nuts and seeds.

Good fats help to optimize your overall health by lowering bad cholesterol and increasing good cholesterol.

Increased fiber consumption

The DASH diet recommends increasing your fiber consumption by eating several servings of fruits, vegetables and grains every day. This keeps you feeling full and it helps to reduce blood pressure.

High fiber consumption also helps to maintain good blood sugar levels and it also encourages weight loss.

Reduction of alcohol and caffeine

The DASH diet suggests limiting your intake of alcohol, soda, tea and coffee because they offer no nutritional value, typically contain a lot of sugar and they can elevate blood pressure.

Customized sodium and caloric intake

In the same way that you can choose a 2300 mg/day or 1500 mg/day sodium intake DASH diet, you can also choose the most suitable caloric intake level for you. The DASH diet allows you to choose a diet of 1500 to 3100 calories per day.

The caloric intake that you choose will depend on your weight, activity level and whether you have high blood pressure now or want to prevent it.

If you are overweight you will likely opt for the lower caloric intake level. If you are active then you will probably choose the higher caloric intake level.

If you have high blood pressure or are at risk of developing high blood pressure due to family history etc. then you'll likely opt for the low sodium diet.

Consider working with your doctor to come up with the best combination of sodium and calorie level for you.

Chapter 4

Dash Diet Food Groups

The DASH diet is easy to follow because it uses common foods that are available at your local grocery store. The DASH diet suggests daily servings for each of the different food groups. The number of servings you eat will depend on your daily calorie needs.

You can have a look at the DASH diet pyramid online if you like by searching "DASH diet pyramid" in "Google images." Choose the pyramid that has a row of 8 glasses of water on the bottom tier. Or you can type in the following link and it will take you straight to it.

http://thedashdiet.net/wp-content/uploads/2013/04/food_pyramid.gif

Please note: The daily servings suggested on the pyramid will vary depending on your calorie needs. You can find the required servings per daily calories in the next chapter on portion control and serving sizes. *

Tier 1 - Water

The highest priority in any diet is making sure that you get the right nutrients. A large part of getting the right nutrients includes consuming enough water through foods and beverages to keep your body working well.

There are many people suffering from dehydration on a regular basis because they don't consume enough fluids to keep their vital organs saturated with water.

The perils of dehydration

60-70% of the human adult body is made up of water. Fat tissue does not contain as much water as lean tissue so the more fat you have on you the harder it is for your body to store the required water needed to help your vital organs function properly.

If one area of your body starts to get dry it reduces the entire flow of fluids within the body. This lowers blood pressure by decreasing the volume of blood flow and it slows the blood pressure against the artery walls.

When this happens, a reduction in the amount of oxygen in the blood occurs. This reduces the oxygen levels reaching the vital organs and body tissue. As this continues, your whole system eventually begins to get unbalanced due to a lack of water.

Every cell in your body is affected by a lack of water. Yet water is lost every day through your breath, urine, perspiration and bowel movements.

When you sweat, you also lose electrolytes, potassium, sodium and chloride which are all essential to a well functioning body.

This is why it's important to replenish your water supply by consuming foods and drinks that contain water.

Thirst is not the first sign of dehydration. By the time you get thirsty or experience a dry mouth your cells are already eagerly craving water.

Headaches, dizziness, an inability to focus and fatigue are all potential signs of dehydration.

To determine whether you are dehydrated, have a look at your urine. It should be clear. If it is yellow or a yellow/orange color then that is a clear sign that you need to consume more water.

How much water do you need?

US News and World Report ran an article in 2013 entitled "The Truth About How Much Water You Should Really Drink." This article stated that in order to determine how much water your body needs, you must first calculate how much water your body requires at rest.

"At rest" would be considered non-vigorous activities like reading or working at a desk.

In order to calculate this, divide your body weight in half. If you weigh 150 pounds then your body requires 75 ounces of water every day. If you weigh 250 pounds then your body requires 125 ounces every day. If you work out in a day you need to increase that number.

The Institute of Medicine has a general guideline that you can follow in regards to daily water consumption. They recommend that women consume 91 ounces (2.7 liters) of water from foods and beverages every day. Men should consume 125 ounces (3.7 liters) a day.

There are also special cases when it comes to daily recommended water intake. For example those who suffer from kidney stones or chronic urinary tract infections will have to consume more water. The elderly may need to adjust standard recommended amounts and those on certain medications for heart disease, depression and ulcers may also have to adjust these amounts.

How to obtain the required amount of fluids

You can obtain fluids through other liquids besides water though not all liquids are created equal and some can actually harm your body if you drink too much of them. Alcoholic beverages or sodas are a couple examples of fluids that can harm your body. Milk, on the other hand is a decent source of fluid that can help keep you hydrated. It comes in second to water.

It is also possible to get some of your water intake from fruits, vegetables and the foods you eat. Watermelon for example is 90 percent water and can help your body stay hydrated.

The core of the DASH diet pyramid is water. A great way to make your H2O intake more appealing is to add lemon to your water along with a drop or two of liquid Stevia.

Signs of dehydration

If you go for an eight hour period of time without emptying your bladder you are dehydrated.

Signs of dehydration include dark urine, feeling tired, cranky, moody and experiencing headaches. When you are dehydrated your heart also has to work harder to push blood through your veins.

Your body will react negatively when it has to compensate for a lack of fluids so make sure to stay hydrated.

Scheduling your fluid consumption into your day

If you're like me, you might occasionally forget to drink water throughout the day. Luckily there are some great alarms and applications online that can remind you.

Don't let a simple thing like forgetting to drink a glass of water during your busy day cause you another headache. Get plenty of fluids and your body will reward you....plus you will be reducing the stress level on your heart.

Tier 2 - Fortified Cereal, Bread, Rice, Pasta

The second tier of the DASH Diet food pyramid includes fortified cereals, breads, rice and pasta. Whole grain varieties of this food group are best since they provide you with the most nutrients and contain higher levels of vitamins and minerals. They also contain the least amount of processed chemicals like added sugars and dyes.

But what do these foods do for you and how are they going to help you in your weight loss efforts?

Grainy foods provide energy

The grainy food group supports your body's energy level as you exert force during exercise or when you use your mind to figure something out, be it a mathematical question or a personal dilemma.

Grainy foods keep you feeling full longer

Just half a cup of long grain rice along with a stir-fry can keep you feeling full longer than if you didn't include a serving of whole grains with your meal.

Eating oats for breakfast is a great idea because they are a great source of soluble fiber. Soluble fiber makes the bowels softer and more able to move your byproducts along better.

Breads contain insoluble fiber and act like a bulking agent that helps keep your system regular.

Tier 3 - Vegetables and Fruits

The next group on the Dash Diet Pyramid includes both vegetables and fruits. The starchier the vegetable the faster it makes you feel full and the longer your feeling of fullness lasts.

The downside to starchy vegetables is that they turn into sugar when processed and often contain less water content than other types of vegetables. Make sure to monitor the serving sizes so you don't eat too many servings of starchy vegetables.

On the other side of the DASH diet pyramid is the fruit section. Rich, sweet and delicious fruits can offer additional water to your diet. They also fill a natural craving for sweetness.

Fruits and vegetables are a great source of phytonutrients and phytochemicals.

Fruits and vegetables are a terrific source of vitamins and minerals that provide your body with the nutrients it needs to fight illnesses and rejuvenate your system. Your body's source of phytonutrients and phytochemicals comes from this food group.

Phytonutrients and phytochemicals are power nutrients that protect you from hypertension as well as several other diseases like diabetes, stroke, heart disease and some cancers.

Fruits and vegetables also help you maintain a healthy weight as they lower cholesterol and blood pressure levels.

Eat colorful fruits and vegetables

Eat fruits and vegetables in an array of colors. Think "rainbow." An acronym that can help you remember the colors of the rainbow is ROY G BIV. This stands for **R**ed, **O**range, **Y**ellow, **Green**, **B**lue, **I**ndigo and **V**iolet – all the colors of the rainbow!

The brighter and more variant the colors, the more nutrients you will get from the fruits and vegetables.

Eating more than the recommended servings

If you choose to eat more than the daily recommended serving (see Chapter 5 for recommended servings) then it's best to eat more vegetables first then migrate to fruits, keeping in mind that some fruits will turn into sugar in your body after you eat them.

When you are deficient in a certain vitamin or mineral there is a vegetable or fruit available that contains the exact nutrient that you need in order to correct that deficiency. Adding a vegetable or fruit to your diet that you may not normally eat will allow you to cover all your nutrient bases so that you can correct your deficiency naturally rather than with a supplement.

Know how to cook your fruits and vegetables

Learning how to cook your fruits and vegetables in order to obtain the most nutrients from them is important.

The loss of nutrients during the cooking process can vary with fruits and vegetables. For example, cooking tomatoes is different than cooking other vegetables because the tomatoes nutrient values increase the longer they are cooked. Other vegetables lose most of their nutrient value when they are cooked for longer periods.

Burning or cooking vegetables on high heat also causes them to lose a lot of their nutrient value. On the other hand, allowing a garlic clove or onion to rest a few minutes after it's been chopped can increase its nutrient value.

It's good to do some research on how to cook vegetables and fruits in order to get the most nutrients from the food you eat.

Tier 4a - Milk, Yogurt, Cheese

The next tier of the DASH diet pyramid includes milk, yogurt and cheese. It shares the level with meat, poultry, fish, dry beans and nuts.

The benefits of dairy

Dairy products are beneficial because they:

Help build stronger teeth and bones

Assist the nervous system in sending and receiving messages

Help muscles squeeze and relax

Help in releasing hormones and other chemicals in the body

Help maintain a normal heartbeat

Calcium is a key ingredient in most dairy products. It is also an important mineral that is involved in all of these bodily functions.

Tier 4b - Fish, Poultry, Dry Beans and Nuts

The next tier of the DASH diet pyramid is the meat, poultry, fish, dry beans, eggs and nuts group. This food group supplies the body with protein, iron, zinc and some vitamin B and it keeps the body healthy and strong.

Always choose lean cuts of meat and remove the skin from meats like chicken and turkey.

Benefits of this food group

Eggs are a great source of iron and protein so that's why they are listed with meats. Most of the fat in an egg comes from the yolk so take that into consideration when deciding how many eggs to eat in one sitting.

Beans are a low-fat source of protein. They also contain a high level of fiber.

Nuts are a great source of iron and protein and they also contain high levels of good fat.

Tier 5 - Fats, Oils, Sweets, Supplements

The highest tier on the food pyramid is the fats, oils, sweets and supplements group. Each item in this food group is to be used sparingly. Opposite that is the calcium, vitamin D, vitamin B12 and supplements group.

The DASH diet pyramid suggests adding calcium, vitamin D and vitamin B12 to your daily regimen because most people are lacking in these vitamins and the loss of these vitamins as we age signifies the importance of an added supplement for these specific nutrients.

Choose your oils and fats wisely

When choosing fats and oils you need to choose wisely. Omega-3 and omega-6 fatty acids are called "essential" fatty acids because the body cannot produce them on its own. You can only get them through food. These fats reduce inflammation and protect against heart disease. You obtain these fats mostly from fish, nuts and certain kinds of vegetables.

Processed foods contain a lot of fats and oils as well but these are not the best kinds of fats and oils to consume.

How much fat, carbohydrates, protein and cholesterol does the DASH diet allow?

Total fat - 27 %

Saturated fats - 6 %

Carbohydrates - 55 % of your calories

Protein - 18 % of your calories

Cholesterol - 150 mg

Chapter 5

Portion Control and Serving Sizes

The DASH diet stresses the importance of portion size, eating a variety of foods and consuming the right amount of nutrients.

Often it is not what you eat that is the problem rather it is how much you eat.

Yes...measuring your food so that you eat balanced portions throughout the day of each food group can be a chore but it is important.

So how do you develop the habit of measuring out portions every time you eat?

I started breaking down store bought packages a long time ago and found that I actually repackaged foods in terribly large quantities for mine and my families required serving sizes.

As I repackaged food I would tell myself that I had to make sure I cooked enough and that I had enough for leftovers. I then started watching what we did with the extra servings that I had repackaged.

Typically, we didn't use them for what I had intended and instead ate more than we should have.

It is surprising to discover that what you really need verses what you actually eat are two very different things.

My husband's diagnosis as a diabetic slowly moved us into a new era of eating in our family. His heart attack and insulin challenges which turned into our diet challenges became the primary purpose behind our willingness to adapt new habits.

Learning to read package labels before I purchased foods became very important. Was the food worth eating? In what seemed like a day my value of worth suddenly changed. My eyes began to open to the importance of choosing high nutrient foods rather than foods that offered little to no nutrients.

I started measuring out snacks into portion sizes and repackaging them into Ziploc bags. This worked well because you didn't have to do the math when you wanted a snack. It was already figured out.

I broke down our meat packages into two, three and sometimes four different meal plans rather than making extra in one or two meals. I found that snacks were snacks and meals were meals.

There was a time when my husband would make a double-decker sandwich for a snack! Those days are behind us now and we realize that a snack is just that, a snack.

The best advice I can offer is to start your "portion size repackaging efforts" with the foods you currently have in the pantry, refrigerator and freezer.

When you start reviewing serving sizes there are some things that will undoubtedly surprise you about what a serving size actually is.

Learn about your foods and the processes taken to get them to market. You may find that buying fresh fruit and cutting it yourself allows you to eat more fruit. Why? Because processing includes additives that drive up the calories while reducing serving size. When fruits are canned they often require sugar as a preservative. This shrinks the portion size.

Also, when you purchase yogurt with real fruit the yogurt will contain additional additives that the manufacturer had to add to the yogurt to keep the fruit from spoiling. This is usually a sugar-based syrup of some sort. It's a better choice to buy plain yogurt and add your own fruit.

DASH diet allowable calories and servings

The DASH diet plan suggests the following servings per day of each food group. There are three different caloric levels so servings have been adjusted to suit each level.

1600 Calories a Day

Grains (preferably whole grains or multi grains) = 6 servings

Vegetables = 3 - 4 servings

Fruits = 4 servings

Fat-free or low-fat milk and milk products = 2 - 3 servings

Lean meats, poultry and fish = 3 - 4 (or fewer) servings

Nuts, seeds, legumes = 3 - 4 servings per week

Fats and oils = 2 servings

Sweets and added sugars = 3 or fewer servings per week

2600 Calories a Day

Grains (preferably whole grains or multi grains) = 10 - 11 servings

Vegetables = 5 - 6 servings

Fruits = 5 - 6 servings

Fat-free or low-fat milk and milk products = 3 servings

Lean meats, poultry and fish = 6 servings

Nuts, seeds, legumes = 1 serving

Fats and oils = 3 servings

Sweets and added sugars = up to 2 servings a day but not required

3100 Calories a Day

Grains (preferably whole grains or multi grains) = 12 - 13 servings

Vegetables = 6 servings

Fruits = 6 servings

Fat-free or low-fat milk and milk products = 3 - 4 servings

Lean meats, poultry and fish = 6 - 9 servings

Nuts, seeds, legumes = 1 serving

Fats and oils = 4 servings

Sweets and added sugars = up to 2 servings a day but not required

So....what does one serving look like?

Here are some examples of what one serving of each food group looks like:

Grains

1 serving is equal to:

1 slice whole-wheat bread

1 ounce dry cereal

½ cup cooked rice, pasta or cereal

Vegetables

1 serving is equal to:

1 cup raw leafy green vegetables

½ cup raw or cooked vegetables

½ cup low sodium vegetable juice

Fruits

1 serving is equal to:

1 medium fruit

¼ cup dried fruit

½ cup fresh, canned or frozen fruit

Fat-free or low-fat milk and milk products

1 serving is equal to:

1 cup milk or yogurt

1 ½ ounces of cheese

Lean meats, poultry and fish

1 serving is equal to:

2 – 3 ounces cooked meats, poultry or fish

1 egg

Nuts, seeds and legumes

1 serving is equal to:

1/3 cup nuts

2 Tbsp peanut butter

2 Tbsp seeds

½ cup cooked legumes

Fats and Oils

1 serving is equal to:

1 tsp soft margarine

1 tsp vegetable oil

1 Tbsp mayonnaise

2 Tbsp low-fat salad dressing

Sweets and added sugars

1 serving is equal to:

1 Tbsp sugar

1 Tbsp jam or jelly

½ cup sorbet

1 cup lemonade

Chapter 6
Dash Diet Food List

Vegetables

Low-Glycemic Vegetables

(Make these your first choice)

Avocados

Arugula

Artichokes

Asparagus

Brussels sprouts

Broccoli

Bell peppers

Celery

Cabbage

Cauliflower

Cucumbers

Collard greens

Eggplant

Green beans

Kale

Lettuce *(the darker the leafy green, the better)*

Mustard greens

Mushrooms

Onions

Radishes

Spinach

Snow peas

Swiss chard

Summer squash

Sprouts

Turnip greens

Zucchini

Higher Glycemic Vegetables

(Make these your second choice)

Acorn squash

Butternut squash

Chickpeas

Carrots

English peas

Sweet potatoes

Spaghetti squash

Tomatoes

Not allowed:

White potatoes

Corn

Fruits

Low Glycemic Fruits *(First choice)*

All fruits are allowed

Apricots

Apples

Blackberries

Blueberries

Bananas

Cranberries

Casaba melon

Cantaloupe

Grapes

Guavas

Honeydew melon

Limes

Lemons

Nectarines

Peaches

Papayas

Rhubarb

Raspberries

Strawberries

Watermelons

Higher Glycemic Fruits *(Second choice)*

Cherries

Figs

Grapefruits

Kiwis

Mango

Oranges

Plums

Pears

Pumpkin

Tangerines

Meats and Seafood

All shellfish

All fish (especially oily fish like salmon, sardines etc)

Beef (choose lean roasts and steaks and extra lean ground meat)

Chicken (skinless)

Eggs

Game birds and meats

Lamb (lean)

Pork (lean roasts and steaks)

Turkey (skinless and ground)

Turkey bacon (low sodium)

Not allowed:

Bacon (regular)

Cold cuts packaged and deli meats

Jerky

Sausage

Dairy

Almond milk

Blue cheese

Cheddar and cottage cheese (low-fat)

Cow's milk (1 % and skim)

Cream cheese (low-fat)

Feta-cheese

Greek yogurt

Margarine or butter substitute

Parmesan cheese (high sodium so limit)

Mozzarella cheese

Provolone cheese (low-fat)

Regular yogurt (low-fat)

Ricotta cheese (low-fat)

Soy milk

Sour cream (low-fat)

Swiss cheese

Not allowed:

Full-fat dairy

Butter

Cream

Fats

Almonds

Black walnuts

Brazil nuts

Canola oil

Flaxseed oil

Butter or margarine substitute

Mayonnaise (low-fat)

Pecans

Olives (low-sodium)

Olive oil

Sesame seeds

Sunflower seeds

Not allowed:

Peanut oil, sesame oil and all other vegetable oils

<u>Grains</u>

Almond flour

Brown rice

Barley

Coconut flour

Wheat germ

Whole-grain bread

Whole-grain low carb cold cereal

Whole-grain mixed grain hot cereal

Whole grain pita

Whole-grain thin bagel

Whole-grain steel-cut oats

Whole-grain thin English muffins

Whole-wheat flour

Whole-grain tortillas

Not allowed:

Corn muffins

Corn bread

Corn meal

Oatmeal (instant or flavored)

Sweetened cold cereals

Condiments, Seasonings and "other"

Almond butter

Agave nectar

Coffee

Caesar dressing

Dressing (low sodium or no sodium)

Flaxseed

Flaxseed oil

Herbs

Spices

Hot sauce

Honey

Mustard (not honey mustard)

Preserves (low or no sugar)

Peanut butter (limit)

Jellies (low or no sugar)

Quinoa

Sesame butter

Salsa

Pickles (sour and dill)

Soy sauce (low sodium)

Teriyaki sauce (low sodium)

Tea (hot or cold)

Tomato of spaghetti sauce (no sugar)

Chicken, beef or vegetable broth (low or no sodium)

Vinaigrette

Whey protein powder (no sugar added)

Soy protein powder

Not allowed:

Alfredo sauce (prepared)

Cheese sauce (prepared)

Gravies (prepared)

Mayonnaise (full-fat)

Barbeque, steak and other sauces (low to regular sodium)

Sweet Treats

Dried fruits (no sugar added)

Fudge pops (fat-free)

Frozen fruit bars (no sugar added)

Gelatin ice cream (low-fat)

1 ounce square dark chocolate

Pudding (fat-free)

Popsicles

Sorbet

Sherbet

Chapter 7

The DASH diet and Weight Loss

Although the DASH diet was not formally created as a weight loss diet it does promote weight loss. This is due to the DASH diets food groups and guidelines.

The well balanced blend of nutritious low calorie whole foods helps your body drop unnecessary weight.

There are three things about the DASH diet that make it particularly great for weight loss:

Consuming healthy fats and omitting unhealthy fats

High fiber intake

High vitamin C intake

The DASH diet and fats

The average American diet contains a lot of unhealthy fat. Trans fats and saturated fats are extremely unhealthy, high in calories and have low to no nutritional value. They are the number one cause of weight gain on the

Standard American Diet (SAD diet). These fats are extremely limited on the DASH diet.

Healthy plant-based fats and omega-3 fatty acids on the other hand are an important part of the DASH diet and highly encouraged. Good fats are excellent for the body and the waist line!

The DASH diet and fiber

The DASH diet includes a lot of foods that contain soluble and insoluble fiber. A high fiber diet helps you feel full longer, slows the absorption of dietary fiber and sugar in your body and improves digestion. This prevents blood sugar spikes while minimizing carbohydrate and junk food cravings. It also prevents fat from being stored in the abdominal area.

A high fiber diet is excellent for your overall health and weight loss!

The DASH diet and vitamin C

The DASH diet encourages a high consumption of fresh fruits and vegetables that are full of vitamins, minerals and antioxidants. One vitamin that plays a huge role in weight loss is vitamin C.

Vitamin C aids in the elimination of stored fat and it prevents hormonal reactions from occurring that can promote fat storage in the abdomen.

Problem is, vitamin C is easily depleted. Stress is the number one thing that depletes vitamin C. When your body lacks vitamin C it tells your brain that you're under stress. This causes a release of the stress hormone cortisol that is sent out to store fat in the abdomen as a safety measure against the threat of famine.

If you can eliminate stress you can eliminate cortisol from being released. Getting a sufficient amount of vitamin C in your diet can also correct cortisol levels.

Having less cortisol in your system not only means a lower accumulation of newly stored fat, it also lets your body know that you don't need the stored fat that you already have. This equals weight loss!

Because vitamin C is a soluble vitamin that gets eliminated in your urine it's important to eat a sufficient amount of vitamin C daily in order to lose body fat. The high consumption of fruits and vegetables on the DASH diet enables you to keep your vitamin C intake high.

Tips to maximize your weight loss

Choose low-calorie foods

You can lose weight on the DASH diet by eating foods that have fewer calories. The key to losing weight is to burn more calories than you eat in a day.

Exchange sweets and other high calorie foods for low calorie foods like fruits and vegetables. Eat smarter, eat smaller portions, eat slowly and be a smart shopper.

Low-fat frozen yogurt will save you nearly 70 calories when compared to full-fat ice cream. Buy low-fat or fat-free when it is available and cut back on portion size.

If you want a snack, choose fresh fruit rather than a cookie or candy. This will increase your fruit consumption and save you about 80 calories per snack.

Dried fruits are a better choice than chips or pork rinds and will save you about 230 calories per snack.

If you have to buy canned fruit make sure it is packaged in water and not syrup.

Plan ahead

Buy an assortment of vegetables, slice them and take them to work along with a sandwich. This will increase your vegetable consumption and it will help you resist the temptation to grab a bag of chips from the vending machine at lunch. Replacing a bag of chips with vegetables will save you about 120 calories.

Choose healthy snacks

Eat healthy snacks without adding unhealthy seasonings. Try popcorn cooked in olive oil and seasoned with garlic or grated parmesan cheese rather than butter and salt.

Choose water

Drink water with a twist of lemon or lime rather than sodas and sweetened teas.

Adhere to recommended serving sizes

Watch your serving sizes on labels.

Consume less sodium

Sodium will make you retain water and it will cause inflammatory responses throughout your body. You need some sodium but not a lot.

Set a goal to watch your sodium intake and start paying attention to the information on food labels. Prepackaged foods can contain excessive amounts of sodium. Aim to buy foods that do not have salt added to them.

Note: Watch the salt content in canned foods, sauces, tomato juices and prepared foods.

Be creative and exchange salt with exotic spices when cooking meals. Let salt be your last resort.

Go low-fat

Choose lower fat methods of preparing your food such as baking, broiling and grilling. Also, reduce the amount of oil and margarine that you use when cooking and use low-fat condiments.

Be smart about eating out

Do some research on the restaurant that you are going to by looking them up online to see how they prepare their food. View their menu online as well. Look for low sodium foods, low-fat, low calorie and special areas on the menu that offer lighter meal plans. If you do not see them ask your server.

Chapter 8

Tips to Make the Switch to DASH Diet Eating

Ease your way into a DASH diet lifestyle by using these helpful tips.

Change gradually

If you currently only eat one or two servings of fruits and vegetables a day try adding a serving at lunch and one at dinner.

Rather than switching to an "all or nothing" approach to whole grains, start by making one or two of your grain serving's whole grains.

Increasing fruits, vegetables and whole grains gradually will help prevent bloating or diarrhea that may occur if you aren't used to eating a high-fiber diet.

Reward successes and forgive slip-ups

Reward yourself with a nonfood treat for your accomplishments such as renting a movie, purchasing a book or getting together with a friend.

Everyone slips up sometimes especially when learning something new. Remember that changing your lifestyle is a long-term process. Find out what triggered your setback then pick up where you left off.

Make exercise an important part of your DASH diet lifestyle

The DASH diet eating plan will improve your health and make you lose weight all on its own. However, if you make regular exercise a habit you will boost your body's ability to shed unwanted pounds.

When you combine DASH diet eating with a good amount of physical activity (30 minutes/day of moderate exercise) it will also maximize your ability to reduce blood pressure.

Get support if you need it

If you are having trouble sticking to your diet talk to your doctor or dietitian about it. They may be able to offer some tips that will help you.

Chapter 9

Tips to Lower Your Sodium Intake

The foods on the DASH diet are naturally low in sodium so you will likely lower your sodium intake just by eating the required foods.

Here are some other ways that you can reduce your sodium intake:

Don't add salt to the water when preparing rice, hot cereal or pasta

Use sodium-free spices, flavorings or condiments with your food instead of salt

Purchase foods labeled "sodium-free," "low sodium" and "no-salt added"

Rinse canned foods to remove some sodium

Get rid of the salt shaker you normally keep on the dinner table

Read food labels

If you are diligent about reading food labels you might be surprised when you see how much sodium is in processed food. Even foods that you consider healthy can still contain a

69

substantial amount of sodium. A couple examples include canned vegetables and low-fat soups.

How much sodium is in salt?

One teaspoon of table salt contains approximately 2300 mg of sodium and a 2/3 teaspoon of salt contains 1500 mg of sodium!

Adjusting to low sodium foods

If food that you normally consume tastes too bland in the "low-sodium" variety then try making more of a gradual increase to low-sodium foods. Be patient. It can take a few months to get used to low sodium foods.

Chapter 10

Dash Diet Seven-Day Meal Plan

Day 1

Breakfast: (442 Cal Total)

3/4 cup pure shredded wheat (125 Cal)

1 cup low-fat organic milk (100 Cal)

1 banana sliced in the cereal (105 Cal)

1 cup of freshly squeezed orange juice (112 Cal)

1 - 8 ounce glass of water (0 Cal)

Morning Snack: (200 Cal)

1/4 cup walnuts, chopped (200 Cal)

Lunch: (311 Cal)

Grilled chicken breast, boneless small (141 Cal)

2 slices whole wheat or whole grain bread (85 per slice x 2 = 170)

1 tablespoon Dijon mustard (0 Cal)

Salad *(29 Cal)*

1/2 cup cucumber slices (8 Cal)

1/2 cup tomato wedges (16 Cal)

1 teaspoon fat free, low sodium Italian Dressing (5 Cal)

1 – 8 ounce glass of water (0)

Afternoon Snack: *(152 Cal)*

3 tablespoons of plain, nonfat yogurt (22 Cal)

1/4 cup of raisins (130 Cal)

Dinner: *(645)*

3 ounces of beef, top sirloin, about the size of a deck of cards (158 Cal)

1 cup green beans, boiled (44 Cal)

1 small baked potato (145 Cal)

½ tablespoon extra virgin olive oil (60 Cal)

1 small apple for dessert (116 Cal)

1 cup of 1 % milk (122 Cal)

1 - 8 ounce glass of water (0 Cal)

Total calories – 1779

Day 2

Breakfast: *(377 Cal)*

1/2 cup oatmeal (not instant) seasoned with cinnamon (150 Cal)

1 medium banana (105 Cal)

1 cup low-fat 2 % milk (122 Cal)

1 glass of water (0 Cal)

Morning Snack: *(160 Cal)*

1/4 cup sunflower seeds (160 Cal)

Lunch: *(617 Cal)*

3 ounces of chicken in chicken salad (100 Cal)

1 leaf of Romaine lettuce up to 2 cups, cut up in salad (15 Cal)

1 slice of tomato diced in salad (16 Cal)

1 celery stick, up to 1 cup, diced in salad (18 Cal)

1 green onion, diced in salad (10 Cal)

1 tablespoon low-fat mayonnaise added to salad (35 Cal)

2 slices of whole wheat or multi grain bread (180 Cal, one slice is 90 Cal)

1 slice of cheese (66 Cal)

1 cup of cantaloupe chunks (60 Cal)

1 cup of apple juice (117 Cal)

8 ounces of water (0 Cal)

Afternoon Snack: *(152.5 Cal)*

1/4 cup dried apricots (100 Cal)

3 tablespoons Greek yogurt (52.5 Cal)

Dinner: *(356 Cal)*

1 cup of whole wheat spaghetti (174 Cal)

1/2 cup mushrooms (22 Cal)

1/2 cup spaghetti sauce no meat (45 Cal)

3 tablespoons parmesan cheese (63 Cal)

1 cup spinach (7 Cal)

1 medium grated carrot (25 Cal)

2 tablespoon fat-free Italian salad dressing (20 Cal)

Total calories – 1662.5

Day 3

Breakfast: *(449 Cal)*

2 cups pure puffed wheat cereal (100 Cal)

1 medium banana (105 Cal)

1 cup - 2 % low-fat milk (122 Cal)

1 cup freshly squeezed orange juice (122 Cal)

8 ounces of water (0 Cal)

Morning Snack: *(238 Cal)*

3/4 cup Greek vanilla yogurt (170 Cal)

1/4 cup blueberries (21 Cal)

1 tablespoon sunflower seeds, no salt added (47 Cal)

Lunch: *(460 Cal)*

3 oz. grilled flounder fish sandwich (100 Cal)

1 slice of cheese, 2 % milk (45 Cal)

1 whole wheat hamburger bun (200 Cal)

1 large leaf of Romaine lettuce (15 Cal)

1 tablespoon low-fat mayonnaise (35 Cal)

1 medium orange (65 Cal)

8 ounces of water (0 Cal)

Afternoon Snack: *(308 Cal)*

2 large graham crackers (118 Cal, each large rectangle or 2 squares is 59 Cal Ea.)

2 tablespoons peanut butter smooth or crunchy same amount of calories (190 Cal)

Dinner: *(248 Cal)*

3 oz. fresh tuna (118 Cal)

1 teaspoon lemon juice (22 Cal)

1 cup cooked spinach (41 Cal)

1 bran muffin (67 Cal)

8 ounces of water (0 Cal)

Total calories – 1703

Day 4

Breakfast: *(404 Cal)*

1 cup Greek yogurt with blueberries (80 Cal)

1 medium peach (40 Cal)

1 slice of wholegrain toast (69 Cal)

1 teaspoon unsalted low-fat margarine (45 Cal)

8 oz. glass 100 percent pure purple grape juice (170 Cal)

8 ounces of water (0 Cal)

Morning Snack: *(281 Cal)*

1 oz. or 24 almonds (164 Cal)

1 cup apple juice (117 Cal)

Lunch: *(316 Cal)*

Ham and cheese sandwich - 2 ounces of ham sliced extra lean 5 percent fat (60 Cal) and 1 slice of 2% cheese (45 Cal) = (105 Cal)

2 slices of whole grain bread for the sandwich (120 Cal)

1 large leaf of Romaine lettuce (15 Cal)

2 slices of tomato (16 Cal)

1 teaspoon low-fat mayonnaise (35 Cal)

1 medium carrot, cut into sticks (25 Cal)

8 ounces of water (0 Cal)

Afternoon Snack: *(139 Cal)*

1 apricot (17 Cal)

1 cup low-fat 2% milk (122 Cal)

Dinner: *(585 Cal)*

Chicken breast skinless, boneless (150 Cal)

3/4 cup brown rice, medium grain (150 Cal)

1 cup green peas boiled in water (124 Cal)

4 oz. cantaloupe chunks (39 Cal)

1 cup low-fat 2% milk (122 Cal)

Total calories – 1725

Day 5

Breakfast: *(669 Cal)*

3/4 cup pure shredded wheat (125 Cal)

1 medium banana (105 Cal)

1 bagel (110 Cal)

1 tablespoon of peanut butter for the bagel (95 Cal)

1 cup low-fat 2% milk (122 Cal)

1 cup orange juice (112 Cal)

8 ounces of water (0 Cal)

Morning Snack: *(94 Cal)*

2 tablespoons of sunflower seeds, unsalted (94 Cal)

Lunch: *(565 Cal)*

2 oz. tuna, solid white albacore (70 Cal)

1 teaspoon low-fat mayonnaise (35 Cal)

1 leaf Romaine lettuce (15 Cal)

1 slice whole grain or whole wheat bread (85 Cal)

Cucumber salad = 1 cucumber (8 Cal)

.....1/2 cup tomato wedges (16 Cal)

.....2 tablespoon red wine vinaigrette (70 Cal)

.....4 oz - 2% low-fat cottage cheese (102 Cal)

.....1 oz. almonds, unsalted (164 Cal)

8 ounces of water (0 Cal)

Afternoon Snack: *(91 Cal)*

1 cup low-fat yogurt strawberry (91 Cal)

Dinner: *(551 Cal)*

4 ounces turkey meatloaf (120 Cal)

1 small baked potato (129 Cal)

1 tablespoon 2% low-fat shredded cheddar (80 Cal)

1 cup collard greens (49 Cal)

1 small whole grain or whole wheat roll (114 Cal)

1 medium peach (59 Cal)

8 ounces of water (0 Cal)

Total calories - 1970

Day 6

Breakfast: (417 Cal)

1 low-fat granola bar - (110 Cal)

1 medium banana (105 Cal)

1 cup low-fat strawberry banana yogurt (80 Cal)

1 cup 2% low-fat milk (122 Cal)

8 ounces water (0 Cal)

Morning Snack: (160 Cal)

1/4 cup sunflower seeds (160 Cal)

Lunch: (404 Cal)

3 ounces of cooked chicken (100 Cal)

2 slices of whole wheat bread (138 Cal - 69 Cal ea.)

1 leaf of Romaine lettuce (15 Cal)

2 slices of tomato (16 Cal)

2 teaspoons low-fat mayonnaise (70 Cal - 35 Cal ea.)

1 orange (65 Cal)

8 ounces of water (0 Cal)

Afternoon Snack: *(17 Cal)*

1 fresh apricot (17 Cal)

Dinner: *(395 Cal)*

1 fillet - trout, wild (215 Cal)

1 cup cooked spinach (41 Cal)

1 carrot (25 Cal)

1 small whole wheat dinner Roll (114 Cal)

8 ounces water (0 Cal)

Total calories - 1393

Day 7

Breakfast: *(341 Cal)*

1/2 cup oatmeal - 150 Cal w/cinnamon to spice = 6 Cal (150 + 6 Cal = 156 Cal)

1 medium banana (105 Cal)

1 cup vanilla yogurt (80 Cal)

8 ounces of water (0 Cal)

Morning Snack: *(164 Cal)*

1 oz. almonds, unsalted (164 Cal)

Lunch: *(443 Cal)*

2 ounces solid white albacore tuna sandwich (70 Cal)

1 tablespoon low-fat mayonnaise (35 Cal)

1 large leaf lettuce (15 Cal)

2 slices of tomato (16 Cal)

2 slices whole wheat bread (120 Cal - 1 slice is 60 Cal)

1 orange (65 Cal)

1 cup 2% low-fat milk (122 Cal)

8 ounces water (0 Cal)

Afternoon Snack: *(182 Cal)*

7 whole wheat crackers (120 Cal)

1 cup purple grapes or white seedless grapes (62 Cal)

Dinner: *(478 Cal)*

3 ounces blackened shrimp skewer - no salt (101 Cal)

Salad = 1 cup fresh spinach (7 Cal)

1 cup tomato wedges (16 Cal)

2 tablespoons red wine vinaigrette (70 Cal)

1 whole wheat or multi grain roll (114 Cal)

8 ounces grape juice (170 Cal)

8 ounces water (0 Cal)

Total calories - 1608

Chapter 11

DASH Diet 30 MINUTE RECIPES

The following recipes are taken from my DASH Diet Recipes book on Amazon

BREAKFAST
Raspberry Muffins

Raspberries contain a phytonutrient called rheosmin also referred to as the raspberry ketone (pronounced key-tone). Studies have found that this enzyme has the ability to accelerate weight loss. Enjoy this nutrient-rich, guilt-free muffin that tastes great and helps you lose weight!

Serves 12

Ingredients

Raspberries.....2/3 cup

Rolled oats.....1/2 cup

1 % low-fat milk.....1 cup

All-purpose flour.....3/4 cup

Grits.....1/4 cup

Wheat bran.....1/4 cup

Baking powder.....1 tablespoon

Salt.....1/4 teaspoon

Dark honey.....1/2 cup

Olive oil.....3 1/2 tablespoons

Lime zest.....2 teaspoons grated

Egg.....1 lightly beaten

Directions

Preheat the oven to 400 °F (200 °C). Line a 12-cup muffin pan with wax paper or foil liners.

In a medium saucepan combine the oats and milk. Cook on medium heat and stir until the oats are tender and the mixture is creamy. Remove from heat and set aside while proceeding to the next step.

In a large bowl combine the flour, grits, bran, baking powder and salt. In a small bowl whisk the eggs and set aside.

Add the honey, olive oil and lime zest to the oats mixture and mix all the ingredients together. Add the egg to the batter. Mix the batter until moistened but still slightly lumpy. Gently fold in the raspberries.

Use two tablespoons, one to scoop the batter and the other to push the batter into the muffin cups, filling each cup about 2/3 full.

Bake until the tops are golden brown. About 16 to 18 minutes. You should be able to insert a toothpick through the center and have it come out clean. If dough sticks to the toothpick, return the muffins to the oven for another minute or two. Transfer the muffins to a wire rack and let them cool completely before serving.

Nutritional analysis per serving

Serving size: 1 muffin

Total carbohydrate 27 g

Dietary fiber 2 g

Sodium 126 mg

Saturated fat 0.5 g

Total fat 5 g

Trans fat <0.5

Cholesterol 16 mg

Protein 3 g

Monounsaturated fat 3 g

Calories 165

Sugars 11 g

Buckwheat Pancakes with Strawberries

Buckwheat is actually a fruit seed and not a cereal grain. It is related to the rhubarb and sorrel family which makes it a great substitute for people who have allergies to wheat or other grains.

Serves 6

Ingredients

Egg whites.....2

Olive oil.....1 tablespoon

Fat-free milk.....1/2 cup

All purpose flour.....1/2 cup

Buckwheat flour.....1/2 cup

Baking powder.....1 tablespoon

Sparkling water.....1/2 cup

Fresh strawberries.....3 cups sliced

Directions

In a large bowl whisk together the egg whites, olive oil and milk.

In another bowl combine the all-purpose flour, buckwheat flour and baking powder and mix thoroughly.

Slowly add the dry ingredients to the egg white mixture as you alternately add the sparkling water. Make sure to mix between each addition until all the ingredients combine into a batter.

Place a nonstick frying pan or griddle over medium heat. Spoon 1/2 cup of the pancake batter into the pan. Cook until the top surface of the pancake bubbles and the edges turn lightly brown, about 2 minutes. Flip and cook until the bottom is nicely brown and cooked through, 1 to 2 minutes longer. Repeat with the remaining pancake batter.

Transfer the pancakes to individual plates. Top each with 1/2 cup sliced strawberries. Serve.

Nutritional analysis per serving

Serving size: 1 pancake

Total carbohydrate 24 g

Dietary fiber 3 g

Sodium 150 mg

Saturated fat - trace

Total fat 3 g

Cholesterol - trace

Protein 5 g

Monounsaturated fat 2 g

Calories 143

Sun-Dried Tomato Basil Pizza

Sun-dried tomatoes have high levels of antioxidants, lycopene and vitamin C. They are often used for tomato paste and tomato purees. The red plum tomato is used for sun-dried products.

Serves 4

Ingredients

12 inch prepared pizza crust purchased or made from mix.....1 crust

Garlic cloves.....4

Fat-free ricotta cheese.....1/2 cup

Dry packed sun-dried tomatoes.....1/2 cup chopped

Dried basil.....2 teaspoons

Thyme.....1 teaspoon

Red pepper flakes

Parmesan cheese

Directions

Preheat the oven to 475 °F (250 °C).

Lightly coat a 12-inch round pizza pie baking pan with cooking spray.

Sun-dried tomatoes need to be reconstituted before using. Place them in a bowl and pour boiled water over them until they are covered in water. Let stand for 5 minutes or until soft and pliable. Drain and chop.

Place the pizza crust in a round pizza pie-baking pan. Arrange garlic, cheese and tomatoes on top of the pizza crust. Sprinkle basil and thyme evenly over the pizza.

Bake on the lowest rack of the oven until the pizza crust turns brown and the toppings are hot, about 20 minutes.

Cut the pizza into eight even slices and serve immediately.

Place the red-flaked pepper jar and the parmesan jar out for individual use.

Nutritional analysis per serving

Serving size: 2 slices

Total fat 2 g

Calories 179

Protein 8 g

Cholesterol 8 mg

Total carbohydrate 32 g

Dietary fiber 2 g

Monounsaturated fat 0.5 g

Saturated fat - trace

Sodium 276 mg

Chicken in White Wine and Mushroom Sauce

Chicken is a great source of protein. For every 100 grams of chicken, you get 30 grams of protein. In comparison, for every 100 grams of tuna, salmon, and halibut there are 26 grams of protein.

This tasty dish is great when served over pasta. Add a side of freshly steamed vegetables for a nutrient rich, delicious meal.

Serves 4

Ingredients

Boneless skinless chicken breast.....4 - 4 ounces each

Olive oil.....2 tablespoons

Shallots.....4 thinly sliced

Fresh mushrooms.....1/4 pound thinly sliced

All-purpose (plain) flour.....1 tablespoon

White wine.....1/4 cup

Chicken stock.....1/2 cup low sodium

Fresh rosemary.....1 tablespoon (or 1 teaspoon dried rosemary)

Fresh parsley.....2 tablespoons chopped

Directions

Place the chicken breasts in a sealed Ziploc bag and pound with a mallet or use a rolling pin to flatten. Remove chicken and cut each piece in half lengthwise. Return to Ziploc bag and refrigerate until firm. When chicken is firm, get two frying pans ready to cook by placing one teaspoon of olive oil in each pan.

In a small bowl add the flour and wine then whisk until all the flour lumps are gone. Set aside.

Turn both of the frying pans to medium heat. In frying pan number one add the chicken breast. In frying pan number two, sauté the shallots for about 3 minutes. Return to frying pan number one and turn the chicken breast over. Go back to frying pan number two and add the mushrooms to the shallots. Stir while the two sauté together for another 2 minutes.

Get the bowl of mixed flour and wine. Whisk a few times and pour over the mushrooms and shallots. Add the chicken stock and stir.

The chicken in the first pan should be a nice shade of brown on each side and cooked through with no pink remaining. Remove from heat and plate. Go back to the mushroom and shallot pan and stir, making sure it has thickened nicely. Turn off the burner and spoon mixture over the chicken. Sprinkle with parsley and serve piping hot.

Nutritional analysis per serving

Serving size: 2 chicken breast halves

Total fat 9 g

Calories 239

Protein 28 g

Cholesterol 66 mg

Total carbohydrate 6 g

Dietary fiber 0.5 g

Monounsaturated fat 5 g

Saturated fat 1 g

Sodium 98 mg

DINNER

Balsamic Chicken Salad with Pineapple

The chicken in this dish provides a great source of protein while the pineapple contains free radicals that fight colds, strengthen bones and improve gums. Pineapple also has anti-inflammatory properties as well as antioxidants for a healthy heart. The nutritional value of pineapple also includes immunity-boosting vitamin C as it prevents hypertension.

Serves 8

Ingredients

Boneless skinless chicken breast..... 4 - each about 5 ounces

Olive oil.....1 tablespoon

Unsweetened pineapple chunks.....1-8 ounce can drained except for 2 tablespoons of juice

Broccoli florets.....2 cups

Fresh baby spinach leaves.....4 cups

Red onions.....1/2 cup thinly sliced

For vinaigrette:

Olive oil.....1/4 cup

Balsamic vinegar.....2 tablespoons

Sugar.....2 teaspoons

Cinnamon.....1/4 teaspoon

Directions

Heat the oil in a large nonstick frying pan on medium heat.

Cut each chicken breast into cubes.

Add the chicken to the heated olive oil and cook until golden brown, about 10 minutes.

In a large serving bowl combine the cooked chicken, sliced onions, pineapple chunks, broccoli and spinach.

Vinaigrette:

Whisk together the olive oil, vinegar and reserved pineapple juice. Add the sugar and cinnamon. Mix together then pour over the salad and gently toss to coat evenly. Serve immediately.

Nutritional analysis per serving

Total carbohydrate 8 g

Dietary fiber 2 g

Sodium 75 mg

Saturated fat 1 g

Total fat 9 g

Cholesterol 41 mg

Protein 17 g

Monounsaturated fat 6 g

Calories 181

Roasted Salmon with Chives and Tarragon

Salmon contains B3, B6, B12 selenium, protein, phosphorus, choline, pantothenic acid, biotin, and potassium. These nutrients are all essential for a healthy cardiovascular system, healthy joints, eye health and a decreased risk of cancer.

Serves 2

Ingredients

Organic salmon with skin.....2 - 5 ounce pieces

Extra virgin olive oil.....2 teaspoons

Chives.....1 tablespoon chopped

Fresh tarragon leaves.....1 teaspoon

Cooking spray

Directions

Preheat the oven to 475 °F (250 °C).

Line a baking sheet with foil and light cooking spray.

Rub salmon all over with 2 teaspoons of extra virgin olive oil.

Roast skin side down about 12 minutes or until fish is thoroughly cooked.

Use a metal spatula to lift the salmon off the skin. Place salmon on serving plate. Discard skin. Sprinkle salmon with herbs and serve.

Nutritional analysis per serving

Total carbohydrate - trace

Dietary fiber - trace

Sodium 62 mg

Saturated fat 2 g

Total fat 14 g

Cholesterol 78 mg

Protein 28 g

Monounsaturated fat 7 g

Calories 241

Triple Berry Spinach Salad

Spinach contains phytonutrients like all other plants but it also contains over a dozen different flavonoid compounds.

There are three classes of flavonoids also known as bioflavonoids. The three classes are flavonoids, isoflavonoids and neoflavonoids. The classes represent the different molecular structures within the flavonoid family.

The flavonoids play a major role in reducing various cardiovascular diseases. They also have antibacterial properties.

Serves 4

Ingredients

Fresh spinach.....4 packed cups, torn

Fresh strawberries.....1 cup sliced

Fresh or frozen blueberries.....1 cup

Sweet onion.....1 small sliced

Pecans......1/4 cup chopped toasted

Salad Dressing:

White wine vinegar or cider vinegar.....2 tablespoons

Balsamic vinegar.....2 tablespoons

Honey.....2 tablespoons

Dijon mustard.....2 teaspoons

Curry powder.....1 teaspoon

Freshly ground black pepper.....1/8 teaspoon

Directions

In a large salad bowl, toss together the spinach, strawberries, blueberries, onion and pecans.

In a small bowl combine the white wine vinegar or cider vinegar, balsamic vinegar, honey, Dijon mustard, curry powder and pepper. Whisk until well mixed.

Drizzle the dressing over the salad then toss to coat. Serve immediately.

Nutritional analysis per serving

Total carbohydrate 25 g

Dietary fiber 4 g

Sodium 197 mg

Saturated fat 0.5 g

Total fat 5 g

Cholesterol 0 mg

Protein 4 g

Monounsaturated fat 3 g

Calories 158

Simple Mango Salad

Mangos help to fight against different types of cancers. They contain vitamin A, beta-carotene, alpha-carotene, beta-cryptoxanthin, potassium, vitamin B6, C, E, and copper.

You can serve this salad over roasted chicken, chicken salad, oriental vegetables, tortellini salads or any salad that can use a little pizzazz!

Serves 6

Ingredients

Mangos.....3 pitted and cubed

Lime.....1 juiced

Red onion.....1 teaspoon minced

Jalapeno pepper.....1/2 seeded and minced

Directions

Combine all the ingredients in a mixing bowl. Cover and place in the refrigerator for 10 minutes. Toss just before serving.

Nutritional analysis per serving

Total carbohydrate 19 g

Dietary fiber 2 g

Sodium 10 mg

Saturated fat - trace

Total fat - trace

Cholesterol 0 mg

Protein 1 g

Monounsaturated fat - trace

Calories 75

APPETIZERS
Tomato Basil Bruschetta

Tomatoes are a terrific choice if you are trying to lose weight. They are also beneficial in cancer prevention. One interesting thing about the tomato is that the more you cook it the higher the nutrient value climbs. Most fruits and vegetables lose their full level of nutritional value when cooked for longer periods but not the tomato!

Serves 6

Ingredients

Whole grain baguette.....1/2 cut into six 1/2 inch thick diagonal slices

Fresh basil......2 tablespoons chopped

Fresh parsley.....1 tablespoon chopped

Garlic cloves.....2 minced

Tomatoes.....3 diced

Fennel.....1/2 cup diced

Olive oil.....1 teaspoon

Balsamic vinegar.....2 teaspoons

Freshly ground black pepper.....1 teaspoon

Parmesan cheese......3 tablespoons

Directions

Dice the tomatoes and place them in a medium bowl. Add chopped basil, parsley, minced garlic, diced fennel, olive oil, balsamic vinegar and black pepper. Stir. Place in the refrigerator for 20 minutes to let the flavors blend.

Preheat the oven to 400 °F (200 °C).

Take the whole grain baguette and cut it into thick diagonal slices about 1/2 inch thick. Set on a baking sheet and put it into the oven. Toast the baguettes until they are lightly browned. Sprinkle with parmesan cheese while hot out of the oven. Transfer to a salsa serving platter.

Add the tomato basil mixture to the platter in a serving bowl with a spoon. Serve immediately.

Nutritional analysis per serving

Serving size: 1 slice

Total carbohydrate 20 g

Dietary fiber 4 g

Sodium 123 mg

Saturated fat < 0.5 g

Total fat 2 g

Trans fat 0 g

Cholesterol 0 mg

Protein 3 g

Monounsaturated fat 1 g

Calories 110

Sugars 0 g

Fruit Kebabs with Lemony Lime Dip

Pineapples have numerous benefits. They prevent free radicals from forming, they have anti-inflammatory and anti-cancer benefits and they help to prevent atherosclerosis.

Strawberries are full of nutrients and can decrease the risk of developing Type-2 diabetes.

Kiwi has phytonutrients that protect DNA. Kiwi is also a good source of fiber as well as other nutrients.

Potassium is a well-known benefit of the banana.

Red grapes offer a whole list of heart-healthy nutrients that include lowering blood pressure and cholesterol levels.

Serves 2

Ingredients

Low-fat sugar-free lemon yogurt.....4 ounces

Lime.....1 for 1 teaspoon lime juice

Lime zest.....1 teaspoon

Pineapple chunks.....4 to 6

Kiwi.....1 peeled and diced

Banana.....1/2 cut into 1/2-inch chunks

Red grapes.....4 to 6

Wooden skewers.....4

Directions

In a small bowl whisk together the lemon yogurt, lime juice and lime zest. Cover and refrigerate to allow the flavors to marinate as you prepare the rest of the recipe.

Thread one of each fruit onto a skewer. Repeat with the other skewers until the fruit is gone. Since Kiwi acts as a natural tenderizer place it next to the pineapple or grapes and avoid setting it right next to the banana to prevent premature browning.

Serve with the lemony lime dip.

To prevent fruit from browning, dip it in pineapple or orange juice.

Nutritional analysis per serving

Serving size: 2 fruit kebabs

Total fat 1 g

Calories 160

Protein 4 g

Cholesterol 4 mg

Total carbohydrate 36 g

Dietary fiber 4 g

Monounsaturated fat - trace

Saturated fat < 1 g

Sodium 45 mg

SAUCES, DRESSINGS AND DIPS

Artichoke Dip

Artichokes are great for calming the stomach or relieving stomach pains. Research has also found that artichokes can help reduce high cholesterol. If you have gallstones check with your doctor before eating artichokes. If you have allergies to ragweed, chrysanthemums, marigolds or daises you should check with your doctor as well since artichokes come from the same family of flowers.

Serves 8

Ingredients

Artichoke hearts.....2 cups

Spinach.....4 cups chopped

Thyme.....1 teaspoon minced

Garlic.....2 cloves minced

Fresh parsley.....1 tablespoon minced

White beans.....1 cup prepared

Parmesan cheese.....2 tablespoons

Low-fat sour cream.....1/2 cup

Freshly ground black pepper.....1 tablespoon

Directions

Preheat the oven to 350 °F (175 °C)

Mix the ingredients together in a large bowl. Transfer to a glass or ceramic dish and bake for 20 minutes.

Serve warm with whole-grain bread, crackers or vegetables for dipping.

Nutritional analysis per serving

Serving size: Approx 1/2 cup

Total carbohydrate 14 g

Dietary fiber 6 g

Sodium 71 mg

Saturated fat 1 g

Total fat 2 g

Trans fat 0 g

Cholesterol 6 mg

Protein 5 g

Monounsaturated fat 1 g

Calories 94

Sugars 0 g

Peach Honey Spread

Peaches are full of vitamins, minerals, protein and beta-carotene that help prevent cancer. The fiber content of peaches assists with healthy digestion. The peach alkaline levels aid in the relief of digestive abnormalities and peaches also contain properties that bring down cholesterol levels.

This tasty spread is great with pancakes, waffles, roasted pork, roasted chicken and even on toast!

Serves 6

Ingredients

Fresh cranberries.....1 cup chopped

Unsweetened peach halves.....1 – 15 ounce can, drained

Honey.....2 tablespoons

Cinnamon.....1/2 teaspoon

Directions

Put the drained unsweetened peach halves in a mixer and set it to chop. When the peaches have a chunky texture comparable to applesauce, transfer them to a large bowl. Add the honey and cinnamon to the peaches. Mix with a large spoon.

Chill in the refrigerator until ready to serve or serve warm over your favorite dish.

Nutritional analysis per serving

Serving size: 1/3 cup

Total fat 0 g

Calories 60

Protein 0.5 g

Cholesterol 0 mg

Total carbohydrate 16 g

Dietary fiber 1 g

Monounsaturated fat 0 g

Saturated fat 0 g

Sodium 4 mg

Other books by Gina Crawford

DASH Diet Recipes

Mediterranean Diet for Beginners

Mediterranean Diet Cookbook

Paleo for Beginners

Sugar Detox for Beginners

Sugar Free Recipes

5 2 Diet for Beginners

5 2 Diet Recipes

Conclusion

Congratulations on finishing the book!

I pour my heart into every book and make every effort to help you achieve your diet and health goals.

I hope this book gave you all the information you needed to understand how to successfully apply the DASH diet to your life TODAY!

May this diet be the beginning of a brand new vibrant you!

About Gina Crawford

Understanding what it takes to live a healthy lifestyle, eat right, achieve your goal weight and love your life shouldn't be complicated. Your time is valuable and the last thing you need is to tackle a 300 page book on how to get your health, weight and life on track. If you're like most people, you just want the facts in bite-sized, easy to understand pieces that you can apply to your life TODAY!

My name is Gina Crawford. I am a health and "all things natural" enthusiast, author, mother and wife. Years ago I was overweight, exhausted, unhappy and desperately aching for a better life. One day, gruelingly tired of my situation, I started researching everything I could on health and transforming my life. Often I felt overwhelmed by the amount of information and the changes I had to make, but I persevered and managed to turn my life around one book and one bite at a time.

Now I'm determined to share what I've learned in an easy, non-overwhelming, "no fluff, no filler, straight to the point" kind of way that will allow others to achieve maximum results in a short amount of time.

I am passionate about every book I write and my goal with each book is to make it simple and concise yet power-packed with the necessary information you need to transform your life. I have learned first-hand the incredible value of healing ourselves with natural organic foods, natural remedies, exercise and a positive mindset.

When I'm not writing, I love spending time with my family, cooking, walking, biking and reading.

My hope is that my books will help you live a healthier, better, more passionate, alive life!

Made in the USA
Lexington, KY
03 August 2015